Lectin Free Diet Guide for Beginners

The Basics of Low-Lectin Alternatives

By

Jamie Kincade

Table of Contents

CHAPTER 1

Introduction

1.1 What Are Lectins?

Lectins are a group of proteins that can be found in a wide variety of foods, particularly in plants, seeds, legumes, and grains. They are part of a plant's natural defense mechanism, serving to protect the plant from predators, such as insects, fungi, and animals. From a botanical perspective, lectins play a crucial role in nature by helping plants survive and propagate. However, when humans consume foods containing high levels of certain lectins, concerns have arisen about their potential impact on health.

Lectins are highly diverse molecules, and they can vary significantly in structure and function. Some lectins have been well-studied and characterized, while others remain less understood. Generally, lectins have an affinity for carbohydrates, and they can bind to specific sugar molecules, such as glucose or mannose. This binding ability is central to their role in plants, as it helps the plant cells interact with other cells, pathogens, and even animals.

The concern surrounding lectins in the human diet stems from the idea that when we consume lectin-rich foods, these lectins can interact with cells in our bodies, particularly in the gastrointestinal tract. Lectins can bind to the lining of the gut, which has led to questions about whether this binding could lead to various health issues.

One of the primary concerns associated with lectins is their potential to disrupt the integrity of the gut lining. This is because lectins have the ability to bind to the surface of the cells in the intestinal lining. Some researchers have suggested that this interaction might compromise the gut barrier, making it more permeable and allowing unwanted substances, such as undigested food particles and toxins, to enter the bloodstream. This concept has given rise to the popular term "leaky gut syndrome."

Proponents of the lectin-free diet argue that reducing or eliminating dietary lectins can help prevent or alleviate various health issues associated with gut health, inflammation, and autoimmune diseases. However, it's important to note that the scientific consensus on this topic is still evolving, and not all experts agree on the extent of the potential risks associated with dietary lectins.

It's also worth mentioning that while lectins are most commonly associated with plant-based foods, they can also be found in some animal products, though in lower concentrations. Therefore, the lectin-free diet primarily focuses on restricting or minimizing the consumption of foods with high lectin content from plant sources.

lectins are naturally occurring proteins in many foods, particularly in plants, seeds, legumes, and grains. They have a carbohydrate-binding ability and have been of interest due to concerns about their potential impact on gut health. The Lectin Free Diet aims to reduce or eliminate these proteins from the diet to address these concerns, although the scientific community continues to explore the extent of the health risks associated with dietary lectins.

CHAPTER 2

Understanding Lectins

2.1 What Are Lectins and Where Are They Found?

What Are Lectins?

Lectins are a class of proteins or glycoproteins found in a wide range of plant and animal foods, although they are more commonly associated with plants. These proteins serve various functions in the biological world, primarily in plants, where they act as a defense mechanism. Lectins are part of a plant's natural immune system, helping protect them against potential threats like insects, fungi, and animals.

Where Are They Found?

Lectins can be found in a variety of foods, and their presence is not limited to any one particular food group. They are most prevalent in:

1. **Legumes:** Beans (e.g., kidney beans, lentils, black beans), peas, and peanuts are well-known sources of lectins. Cooking can significantly reduce lectin content in these foods.

2. **Grains:** Grains such as wheat, rice, and barley contain lectins, primarily in the outer layers or bran. This is one reason why some people following a lectin-free diet opt for alternative grains.

3. **Nightshades:** Vegetables like tomatoes, potatoes, and eggplants are part of the nightshade family and contain lectins. Cooking, especially peeling and deseeding, can help reduce lectin levels in these foods.

4. **Nuts and Seeds:** Almonds, cashews, chia seeds, and sunflower seeds are examples of nuts and seeds that contain lectins. Roasting or soaking can lower lectin levels in some of these foods.

5. **Dairy:** Dairy products like milk and cheese can contain lectins, primarily in the proteins. However, many individuals who follow a lectin-free diet may still consume dairy in moderation, as lectin content is

generally lower compared to some plant-based sources.

6. **Seafood:** Certain seafood, such as shellfish and mollusks, contain lectins. However, the lectin content in seafood is relatively low compared to plants and legumes.

7. **Animal-Based Foods:** While animal-based foods contain lectins in lower concentrations, they are not excluded from a lectin-free diet. It's the plant-based lectin sources that are of greater concern.

It's essential to note that the lectin content in these foods can vary depending on factors like the type of plant or animal, cultivation methods, and food processing techniques. Some proponents of the lectin-free diet recommend careful preparation methods, such as soaking, boiling, and pressure cooking, to reduce lectin levels in high-lectin foods.

2.2 How Do Lectins Impact Health?

The impact of dietary lectins on health is a subject of ongoing research and debate. Some proponents of the lectin-free diet argue that lectins can have negative health effects, particularly when consumed in large quantities, as they can potentially interact with the human body in various ways. Here are some potential ways lectins are believed to impact health, though it's important to note that the scientific consensus on these effects is still evolving:

1. **Gut Health:** One of the primary concerns is that lectins may bind to the lining of the gut, potentially disrupting the integrity of the intestinal barrier. This has led to the concept of "leaky gut syndrome," where the gut becomes more permeable, allowing undigested food particles and other substances to enter the bloodstream. Proponents argue that this may contribute to digestive issues and inflammation.

2. **Inflammation:** Some research suggests that lectins may have pro-inflammatory properties and could trigger an inflammatory response in the body, which, over time, may contribute to chronic

inflammation, a known risk factor for various diseases.

3. **Autoimmune Diseases:** There is a hypothesis that lectins, by interfering with the immune system and potentially promoting inflammation, may play a role in the development or exacerbation of autoimmune diseases.

It's important to stress that these potential negative effects are still a matter of debate and ongoing scientific investigation. Not all experts agree on the extent of the risk, and many factors, including an individual's overall diet, genetic makeup, and gut health, can influence how lectins interact with the body. Some proponents of the lectin-free diet claim health benefits from avoiding high-lectin foods, while others maintain that such a diet may be unnecessarily restrictive. Further research is needed to provide more conclusive evidence on the relationship between lectins and health.

2.3 Lectins and Digestion

Lectins have been the subject of interest and concern regarding their potential impact on digestion. The interaction between lectins and the digestive system is a central aspect of the debate surrounding the lectin-free diet. Here's an overview of how lectins might affect digestion:

Binding in the Gut: Lectins have an affinity for carbohydrates, and they can bind to the lining of the gastrointestinal tract. This binding property is a point of concern for some, as it may lead to various effects, including the following:

- **Impaired Nutrient Absorption:** Some argue that lectin binding to the gut lining could interfere with the absorption of essential nutrients, including vitamins and minerals, potentially leading to nutritional deficiencies.

- **Digestive Discomfort:** The binding of lectins to the gut lining may also result in digestive discomfort, such as gas, bloating, or diarrhea, particularly when high-lectin foods are consumed in large quantities.

- **Leaky Gut Syndrome:** As mentioned earlier, there is a

concept known as "leaky gut syndrome," which suggests that lectins, among other factors, might increase the permeability of the intestinal barrier. This could potentially allow undigested food particles and toxins to enter the bloodstream, contributing to systemic inflammation.

Individual Variation: It's important to note that the effects of lectins on digestion can vary significantly from one person to another. Factors such as an individual's genetic makeup, gut health, and overall diet can influence how lectins interact with the digestive system. Not everyone experiences digestive issues related to lectin consumption, and some individuals may tolerate lectin-containing foods without any problems.

Mitigation Strategies: For those concerned about the potential digestive impact of lectins, there are strategies to mitigate these effects, including soaking, boiling, and fermenting certain high-lectin foods. These processes can reduce lectin content and make foods more digestible.

2.4 Lectins and Inflammation

Another area of concern regarding lectins is their potential to promote inflammation in the body. Chronic inflammation is associated with a range of health problems, including cardiovascular disease, autoimmune conditions, and various chronic diseases. Here's how lectins are thought to be linked to inflammation:

Pro-Inflammatory Properties:
Some research suggests that certain lectins may have pro-inflammatory properties. When lectins interact with the gut lining, immune cells may become activated, leading to an inflammatory response. This inflammation could contribute to chronic low-grade inflammation, which is a risk factor for many health conditions.

Autoimmune Diseases: An extension of the inflammation hypothesis is that lectins may contribute to or exacerbate autoimmune diseases. In autoimmune diseases, the immune system mistakenly attacks the body's own tissues. Some proponents of the lectin-free diet argue that lectins may trigger or worsen autoimmune responses by increasing inflammation and promoting immune system dysfunction.

Research Gaps: It's important to note that the link between lectins and inflammation is an area of ongoing research and debate. While some studies suggest that lectins have inflammatory properties, not all research supports this idea. Additionally, the extent to which dietary lectins contribute to inflammation in the context of a well-balanced diet is still not well-established.

Individual Responses: As with digestion, individual responses to lectins and inflammation can vary. Not everyone who consumes lectin-containing foods will experience increased inflammation, and the impact of lectins may depend on individual factors, including genetics and overall dietary patterns.

The potential impact of lectins on digestion and inflammation remains a subject of scientific investigation and debate. While there are concerns that lectins may bind to the gut lining, disrupt digestion, and promote inflammation, the effects can vary among individuals. Some people may choose to reduce or eliminate high-lectin foods from their diet as a precaution, while others continue to consume them without experiencing negative effects. Further research is needed to better understand the relationship between lectins and health.

CHAPTER 3

The Science Behind the Lectin Free Diet

3.1 Research and Studies

The science behind the lectin-free diet is an area of ongoing research and study, and the available evidence is both limited and somewhat contentious. Here's an overview of the existing research and studies related to the lectin-free diet:

Research Supporting the Diet:

- **Animal and Cell Studies:** Some animal and cell studies have suggested that certain lectins can indeed have adverse effects when consumed in large quantities. These effects may include intestinal damage, inflammation, and autoimmune reactions. These findings have provided some of the scientific basis for concerns about lectin consumption.

- **Small Human Studies:** A handful of small-scale studies in humans have explored the potential impact of dietary lectins on health. These studies have reported associations between lectin consumption and digestive symptoms, such as bloating and gas. However, the sample sizes in these studies have been limited, and more research is needed to draw definitive conclusions.

Criticisms and Limitations:

- **Insufficient Human Research:** A major criticism of the lectin-free diet is the scarcity of robust human studies to support its claims. While animal and cell studies provide some insights, their applicability to humans can be limited. More large-scale, controlled human trials are necessary to determine the true impact of dietary lectins on health.

- **Lack of Consensus:** The scientific community has not reached a consensus on the extent of the potential risks associated with lectins. Critics argue that the diet may be overly restrictive and not grounded in sufficient evidence to warrant the avoidance of lectin-containing foods.

- **Variability in Individual Responses:** Individual responses to lectins can vary widely. While some individuals report digestive discomfort or inflammation after consuming high-lectin foods, others may experience no adverse effects. The reasons behind these differences remain complex and not fully understood.

3.2 Criticisms and Controversies

The lectin-free diet is not without its share of criticisms and controversies. Here are some of the main points of contention:

- **Lack of Scientific Consensus:** One of the primary criticisms of the lectin-free diet is the lack of scientific consensus. Many experts argue that the evidence supporting the diet's claims is limited and inconclusive. Some even consider it to be a fad diet without sufficient scientific backing.

- **Overly Restrictive:** Critics contend that the diet is overly restrictive, eliminating many nutritious foods, such as whole grains, legumes, and certain vegetables, without clear evidence of harm for most individuals. This restriction can make it challenging to obtain a balanced and varied diet, potentially leading to nutritional deficiencies.

- **Potential Nutritional Gaps:** Eliminating lectin-containing foods can create nutritional gaps, as these foods provide essential nutrients like fiber, vitamins, and minerals. Critics argue that individuals following the diet may need to take extra precautions to ensure they get all the nutrients they need.

- **Lack of Long-Term Studies:** Long-term studies on the health effects of the lectin-free diet are limited. It's unclear how the diet may impact health over an extended period, including potential benefits and risks.

3.3 Potential Benefits

Proponents of the lectin-free diet claim various potential benefits, although it's important to recognize that these claims are still a matter of debate and ongoing research. Some of the potential benefits often associated with the diet include:

- **Improved Digestive Health:** Some individuals report relief from digestive discomfort and symptoms, such as bloating and gas, after eliminating high-lectin foods from their diet. For these individuals, the diet may lead to improved digestive health.

- **Reduced Inflammation:** There is some evidence to suggest that lectins can have pro-inflammatory properties. As a result, proponents argue that avoiding high-lectin foods may reduce inflammation, potentially lowering the risk of chronic diseases associated with inflammation.

- **Management of Autoimmune Conditions:** Proponents suggest that the lectin-free diet can be particularly beneficial for individuals with autoimmune conditions. By reducing inflammation and potentially modulating the immune system, the diet may help manage symptoms in some cases.

- **Weight Loss:** Some individuals may experience weight loss when following the lectin-free diet. This can be attributed to reduced calorie intake or changes in food choices.

The science behind the lectin-free diet is an evolving and contentious field. While some studies and anecdotal reports suggest potential benefits, the lack of consensus, limited research in humans, and criticisms about the diet's restrictiveness make it a topic of ongoing debate in the scientific and medical communities. Before adopting the diet, it's crucial to consult with a healthcare professional to weigh the potential benefits against the risks and ensure that nutritional needs are met.

CHAPTER 4

Foods to Avoid on a Lectin Free Diet

4.1 High-Lectin Foods

When following a lectin-free diet, it is essential to be aware of and avoid foods that are high in lectins. High-lectin foods are those that contain significant levels of lectins, and they are the primary targets for exclusion from the diet. Here are some examples of high-lectin foods:

- **Legumes:** Beans, lentils, chickpeas, and peas are notorious for their high lectin content. These foods are a staple source of protein in many diets but are typically avoided on a lectin-free diet. If you choose to include them in your diet, it's recommended to properly prepare them through methods like soaking and cooking to reduce lectin levels.

- **Grains:** Certain grains, such as wheat, barley, and rice, contain lectins, particularly in the bran or outer layers. Whole grains, which are rich in fiber and nutrients, are a common source of lectins, so many lectin-free diets advise avoiding them in favor of alternative grains with lower lectin content.

- **Nightshades:** Vegetables from the nightshade family, including tomatoes, potatoes, eggplants, and bell peppers, contain lectins. These vegetables are staples in many cuisines but are sometimes restricted on a lectin-free diet.

- **Nuts and Seeds:** Some nuts and seeds, such as almonds, cashews, and chia seeds, contain lectins. Roasting, soaking, or processing these foods can help reduce lectin levels.

- **Dairy:** While dairy products generally contain fewer lectins compared to plant-based sources, some individuals following a strict lectin-free diet may choose to limit or avoid dairy altogether. Milk and cheese are examples of dairy products that contain lectins.

- **Processed and Refined Foods:** Many processed and refined foods, including certain grains and legumes, often contain added lectins. Reading food labels and avoiding heavily processed foods is essential for those following a lectin-free diet.

It's important to note that the degree of lectin reduction varies with different preparation methods. Soaking, boiling, and pressure cooking are often recommended to reduce lectin content in high-lectin foods if you choose to include them in your diet.

4.2 Hidden Sources of Lectins

Lectins can also be found in unexpected places, and it's important to be vigilant about hidden sources of lectins when following a lectin-free diet. Here are some examples of potential hidden sources of lectins:

- **Canned Foods:** Some canned foods, especially those not properly prepared or processed, may still contain significant lectin levels. When possible, choose fresh or frozen vegetables over canned options.

- **Condiments and Sauces:** Certain condiments and sauces, such as ketchup and soy sauce, can contain lectins. It's important to check labels and opt for lectin-free alternatives or make homemade versions.

- **Grains in Processed Foods:** Processed foods often contain ingredients derived from grains that are high in lectins. Be cautious of foods like breakfast cereals, bread, and snack bars that may contain lectin-containing grains.

- **Cross-Contamination:** Cross-contamination can occur when high-lectin foods come into contact with other foods during preparation or cooking. To minimize this risk, ensure separate preparation surfaces, utensils, and cookware are used for lectin-free foods.

- **Hidden Ingredients:** Ingredients like modified food

starch, hydrolyzed vegetable protein, and textured vegetable protein are often derived from high-lectin sources. These hidden ingredients can be present in various processed foods, so it's important to scrutinize ingredient lists.

4.3 Cooking and Processing to Reduce Lectins

For those who wish to include high-lectin foods in their diet or reduce lectin levels in certain foods, there are cooking and processing methods that can be employed to minimize lectin content. Here are some techniques:

- **Soaking:** Soaking legumes, grains, nuts, and seeds in water for an extended period (usually overnight) can help reduce lectin levels. Discarding the soaking water before cooking is a common practice to remove lectins.

- **Boiling:** Cooking high-lectin foods at high temperatures, such as boiling, can further reduce lectin content. It's essential to ensure that foods are cooked thoroughly to eliminate lectins.

- **Pressure Cooking:** Pressure cooking is known to be especially effective at breaking down lectins in foods. It can significantly reduce lectin content, making certain high-lectin foods safer for consumption.

- **Peeling and Deseeding:** In the case of nightshades, such as tomatoes and peppers, removing the skin and seeds can help lower the lectin content. However, this may result in nutrient loss as well.

- **Fermentation:** Fermenting certain foods, like sourdough bread, can help break down lectins. Fermentation is a traditional method of food preparation that can make some high-lectin foods more digestible.

a lectin-free diet involves avoiding or minimizing the consumption of high-lectin foods, such as legumes, grains, nightshades, nuts, and seeds. Additionally, it's important to be vigilant about hidden sources of lectins and employ cooking and processing methods like soaking, boiling, and pressure cooking to reduce lectin levels in foods when necessary. These strategies can make the diet more manageable and help ensure the avoidance of potentially problematic lectin-containing foods.

CHAPTER 5

Foods to Include on a Lectin Free Diet

5.1 Low-Lectin Alternatives

While a lectin-free diet involves restricting or avoiding high-lectin foods, there are plenty of low-lectin alternatives that you can incorporate into your meals. These alternatives offer a source of nutrition without the concerns associated with high-lectin foods. Here are some examples of low-lectin alternatives:

- **Protein Sources:** Opt for animal-based proteins such as lean meats (e.g., poultry, fish, and beef), eggs, and dairy (if tolerated). These foods are generally low in lectins and provide essential amino acids.

- **Non-Nightshade Vegetables:** A wide variety of vegetables are low in lectins and suitable for a lectin-free diet. Options include leafy greens, broccoli, cauliflower, carrots, zucchini, and cucumbers.

- **Low-Lectin Fruits:** Many fruits are low in lectins, making them a great addition to a lectin-free diet. Examples include berries, apples, pears, and citrus fruits.

- **Alternative Grains:** If you prefer to include grains in your diet, opt for alternative grains with lower lectin content. Some options include quinoa, rice (especially white rice), and oats.

- **Herbs and Spices:** Most herbs and spices are low in lectins and can add flavor to your dishes without concerns. Examples include basil, oregano, rosemary, and turmeric.

- **Healthy Fats:** Olive oil, avocado oil, and coconut oil are healthy fats that are low in lectins and can be used for cooking and salad dressings.

- **Nuts and Seeds:** While some nuts and seeds are high in lectins, others have lower levels. For example, macadamia nuts, pine nuts, and pumpkin seeds are considered low-lectin options.

- **Dairy (if tolerated):** For those who can tolerate dairy, it can be included in a lectin-free diet. Options like butter and hard cheeses are generally lower in lectins.

5.2 Nutrient-Rich Foods

Incorporating nutrient-rich foods into your lectin-free diet is crucial to ensure you're obtaining essential vitamins and minerals. A balanced diet should provide the necessary nutrients for overall health. Here are some nutrient-rich foods to consider:

- **Leafy Greens:** Greens like spinach, kale, and Swiss chard are packed with vitamins, minerals, and antioxidants, making them valuable additions to your diet.

- **Colorful Vegetables:** Vegetables of various colors, such as red, orange, and purple bell peppers, carrots, and beets, offer a range of nutrients.

- **Berries:** Berries like blueberries, strawberries, and raspberries are rich in antioxidants, fiber, and vitamins.

- **Lean Proteins:** Incorporate lean sources of animal-based proteins like skinless poultry, fish, and lean cuts of meat to provide essential amino acids.

- **Fatty Fish:** Fatty fish such as salmon, mackerel, and sardines are excellent sources of omega-3 fatty acids and other essential nutrients.

- **Nuts and Seeds:** Nutrient-dense options include almonds, walnuts, and chia seeds. These provide healthy fats, protein, and various vitamins and minerals.

- **Eggs:** Eggs are an affordable and nutritious source of protein, vitamins, and minerals.

- **Dairy (if tolerated):** Dairy products like yogurt and hard cheeses can provide calcium and protein.

5.3 Meal Planning and Recipes

Effective meal planning is essential for successfully following a lectin-free diet. It can help you maintain variety in your diet and ensure you're meeting your nutritional needs. Here are some tips for meal planning and finding recipes:

- **Plan Balanced Meals:** Aim for meals that include a source of protein, vegetables, and healthy fats. This will help you obtain a wide range of nutrients and create satisfying, balanced dishes.

- **Use Cookbooks and Online Resources:** There are many cookbooks and online resources dedicated to lectin-free recipes. These can provide inspiration and guidance for preparing delicious and nutritious meals.

- **Meal Prepping:** Consider meal prepping to save time and ensure you have lectin-free meals readily available. You can prepare ingredients in advance and assemble meals for the week.

- **Experiment with Alternative Grains:** While some grains are restricted on a lectin-free diet, you can explore alternative grains like quinoa, rice, and oats for variety in your meals.

- **Explore Lectin-Free Substitutes:** Many lectin-free recipes offer creative substitutes for traditional high-lectin ingredients. For example, cauliflower rice can replace traditional rice in recipes.

- **Keep It Simple:** Not all lectin-free meals need to be elaborate. Simple dishes with fresh, whole ingredients can be both nutritious and satisfying.

- **Consult a Nutritionist:** If you have specific dietary needs or concerns, consider consulting a nutritionist or dietitian who can help you create a customized meal plan.

lectin-free diet can include a wide range of low-lectin foods, nutrient-rich options, and creative recipes.

Effective meal planning and a variety of ingredients will help you maintain a balanced and satisfying diet while adhering to the principles of the diet.

CHAPTER 6

Getting Started on a Lectin Free Diet

6.1 Preparing Your Kitchen

Before you begin a lectin-free diet, it's important to prepare your kitchen to make the transition smoother and set yourself up for success. Here are some steps to help you get started:

- **Purge High-Lectin Foods:**
  Start by identifying and
  removing high-lectin foods
  from your pantry, refrigerator,
  and freezer. This includes items
  like beans, lentils, certain
  grains, and nightshade
  vegetables.

- **Stock Low-Lectin
  Alternatives:** Replace high-
  lectin foods with low-lectin
  alternatives. Ensure you have a
  variety of lectin-free foods on
  hand, such as lean proteins,
  leafy greens, colorful
  vegetables, low-lectin fruits,
  and alternative grains.

- **Check Labels:** When
  purchasing packaged or
  processed foods, carefully read
  ingredient labels to avoid

products containing hidden sources of lectins.

- **Invest in Cooking Equipment:** Consider investing in a pressure cooker or Instant Pot, which can help reduce lectin levels in foods like beans and grains. These devices make meal preparation more convenient.

- **Organize Your Kitchen:** Organize your kitchen with the lectin-free diet in mind. Arrange low-lectin foods in easily accessible locations, and use clear labels for any bulk ingredients to stay organized.

6.2 Creating a Shopping List

Creating a shopping list is an essential part of successfully following a lectin-free diet. It ensures that you have the right ingredients on hand to prepare lectin-free meals. Here are some tips for creating an effective shopping list:

- **Plan Your Meals:** Start by planning your meals for the week. This will help you identify what ingredients you need.

- **Focus on Fresh Foods:** Prioritize fresh, whole foods like lean proteins, vegetables, fruits, and low-lectin grains.

- **Check Your Pantry:** Before heading to the store, review your pantry to see which staple items you may need to restock.

- **Review Recipes:** If you're using specific lectin-free recipes, review them to determine the required ingredients and add them to your list.

- **Stick to Your List:** When shopping, stick to your list to avoid purchasing high-lectin foods on impulse.

- **Explore Alternative Ingredients:** Look for lectin-free alternatives for ingredients you typically use. For example, consider using cauliflower rice instead of regular rice.

- **Consider Special Dietary Needs:** If you have additional dietary restrictions or preferences, such as gluten-free or dairy-free, be sure to account for those when creating your shopping list.

6.3 Meal Prep Tips

Meal preparation can significantly ease the process of following a lectin-free diet and save you time during the week. Here are some meal prep tips:

- **Batch Cooking:** Prepare larger batches of lectin-free foods, such as roasted vegetables, lean proteins, or alternative grains, that you can use in multiple meals throughout the week.

- **Portion Control:** Divide prepared meals into portion-controlled containers to make it easy to grab a ready-made lectin-free lunch or dinner.

- **Prep Ingredients:** Wash, chop, and prepare vegetables and fruits in advance. This makes it convenient to add them to meals.

- **Use Make-Ahead Recipes:** Explore lectin-free make-ahead recipes that can be stored and reheated when needed. These can save you time on busy days.

- **Meal Prepping Tools:** Consider investing in meal prep tools like airtight containers, a slow cooker, or a food processor to simplify the process.

- **Label and Date:** Label containers with the date and

contents to keep track of freshness.

6.4 Dining Out and Traveling

Managing your diet when dining out or traveling can be a challenge, but with some planning and strategies, you can still follow a lectin-free diet successfully:

- **Research Restaurants:** When dining out, research restaurant menus in advance. Many establishments now offer online menus, which can help you identify lectin-free options.

- **Ask Questions:** Don't hesitate to ask restaurant staff about ingredients, preparation methods, and accommodations for dietary restrictions. Most restaurants are willing to cater to specific dietary needs.

- **Customize Your Order:** When dining out, be prepared to customize your order to make it lectin-free. For example, request the removal of nightshade vegetables or grains from a dish.

- **Pack Snacks:** When traveling, carry lectin-free snacks with you to ensure you have suitable options when on the go. Nuts, fresh fruit, and rice cakes can be convenient choices.

- **Research Local Cuisine:** If traveling to a foreign destination, research the local cuisine to identify lectin-free options and familiarize yourself with any potential challenges.

- **Consider Accommodations:** If you have strict dietary requirements, you may opt for accommodations with kitchen facilities when traveling. This allows you to prepare your meals.

Getting started on a lectin-free diet involves preparing your kitchen, creating a shopping list, meal planning, and addressing challenges when dining out or traveling. By taking these steps, you can set yourself up for a successful transition to a lectin-free lifestyle and maintain your dietary goals.

CHAPTER 7

Benefits and Potential Drawbacks

7.1 Potential Health Benefits

A lectin-free diet is a dietary approach that has generated interest for its potential health benefits, although these are still a matter of ongoing research and debate. Here are some potential health benefits often associated with the diet:

- **Improved Digestive Health:** For some individuals, particularly those with specific digestive sensitivities, a lectin-free diet may lead to improved digestive health by reducing symptoms like bloating and gas. By avoiding high-lectin foods, which can be challenging to digest for some, individuals may experience relief.

- **Reduced Inflammation:** Some proponents argue that by eliminating lectins, which can have pro-inflammatory properties, the diet may help reduce overall inflammation. Chronic inflammation is a known risk factor for various diseases, so mitigating it may have health benefits.

- **Potential for Autoimmune Condition Management:** Some people with autoimmune conditions have reported improvements in their symptoms and disease management when following a lectin-free diet. The reduction in inflammation and immune system modulation are potential mechanisms for these benefits.

- **Weight Management:** Weight loss can be an unintended but beneficial side effect of following a lectin-free diet. By eliminating certain high-calorie, high-lectin foods, individuals may reduce their calorie intake and subsequently lose weight.

7.2 Common Concerns

While there are potential benefits associated with the lectin-free diet, it's also essential to consider common concerns and drawbacks:

- **Lack of Scientific Consensus:** A major concern with the lectin-free diet is the lack of scientific consensus. Not all experts agree on the extent of the potential risks associated with dietary lectins, and the scientific evidence supporting the diet's claims is limited and inconclusive.

- **Overly Restrictive:** Critics argue that the diet is overly restrictive, eliminating many nutritious foods. This restriction can make it challenging to obtain a balanced and varied diet, potentially leading to nutritional deficiencies. Avoiding entire food groups, like legumes and grains, may reduce the intake of essential nutrients.

- **Potential Nutritional Gaps:** Eliminating lectin-containing foods can create nutritional gaps, as these foods provide essential nutrients like fiber, vitamins, and minerals. Individuals following the diet may need to take extra precautions to ensure they get all the nutrients they need through other means.

- **Individual Variability:** Individual responses to lectins and the lectin-free diet can vary widely. While some individuals report digestive discomfort or inflammation after consuming high-lectin foods, others may experience no adverse effects. The reasons behind these differences are complex and not fully understood.

- **Difficulty Dining Out and Traveling:** Following a lectin-free diet can be challenging when dining out or traveling. Many restaurant menus and international cuisines may include high-lectin foods, making it necessary to plan ahead and customize your orders.

7.3 Monitoring Your Health

To make an informed decision about whether the lectin-free diet is suitable for you and to mitigate potential drawbacks, it's crucial to monitor your health and make dietary choices that align with your specific needs:

- **Consult a Healthcare Professional:** Before starting a lectin-free diet, consult with a healthcare professional, such as a doctor or registered dietitian, to discuss your individual health goals and dietary needs. They can help you determine if the diet is appropriate for you and provide guidance on maintaining a balanced diet.

- **Regular Health Check-Ups:** If you choose to follow a lectin-free diet, schedule regular health check-ups to monitor your overall health and nutritional status. These check-ups can help identify any potential deficiencies or concerns.

- **Listen to Your Body:** Pay attention to how your body responds to the diet. If you experience adverse effects, such as fatigue, nutritional deficiencies, or other health issues, consult with a healthcare professional and consider modifications to your dietary approach.

- **Customize Your Diet:** While there are common guidelines for a lectin-free diet, you can customize your approach to meet your unique needs. For example, you may choose to reintroduce certain low-lectin foods that you tolerate well.

lectin-free diet offers potential health benefits, but it also raises concerns about its restrictiveness and the lack of scientific consensus. By consulting with healthcare professionals, monitoring your health, and customizing the diet to your specific needs, you can make an informed decision about whether it is the right dietary approach for you.

CHAPTER 8

Tips for Long-Term Success

8.1 Staying Committed

Maintaining a lectin-free diet in the long term requires commitment and consistency. Here are some tips to help you stay committed to your dietary goals:

- **Set Realistic Expectations:** Understand that long-term success may involve occasional setbacks or deviations from the diet. It's essential to have realistic expectations and not be too hard on yourself if you occasionally consume lectin-containing foods.

- **Plan Your Meals:** Meal planning and preparation can be instrumental in staying committed. By having lectin-free meals readily available, you reduce the temptation to veer off the diet.

- **Track Your Progress:** Keep a food journal to monitor your dietary choices and how they impact your health and well-being. This can help you stay motivated and accountable.

- **Celebrate Small Wins:** Celebrate your successes, no matter how small. Recognize and reward yourself for sticking to the diet and meeting your health goals.

- **Stay Informed:** Continue to educate yourself about the latest developments in lectin research and the potential impact of dietary lectins on health. Being well-informed can help you make confident and informed dietary choices.

8.2 Finding Support

Support from friends, family, or a community can be valuable in maintaining a lectin-free diet. Here are some tips for finding and utilizing support:

- **Share Your Goals:** Let your close friends and family know about your dietary choices and the reasons behind them. This can help them understand your needs and provide support.

- **Join Online Communities:** There are online forums and communities where individuals following a lectin-free diet share experiences, tips, and recipes. Participating in these communities can provide a sense of camaraderie and valuable information.

- **Seek Professional Guidance:** Consider working with a registered dietitian or nutritionist who can offer personalized guidance and support. They can help you plan meals, monitor your health, and provide expert advice.

- **Involve Your Household:** If others in your household are also interested in following a lectin-free diet, involve them in meal planning and preparation. This can make the diet a shared and more manageable effort.

- **Be Patient with Others:** Understand that not everyone in your life will share your dietary choices or restrictions. Be patient with friends and family who may not fully grasp your dietary needs.

8.3 Gradual Reintroduction of Foods

While the lectin-free diet involves avoiding or restricting certain foods, some individuals may consider gradually reintroducing certain items to see how they impact their health. Here are some tips for reintroducing foods:

- **Consult with a Professional:** Before reintroducing foods, consult with a healthcare professional or registered dietitian to discuss your plan and monitor your health during the process.

- **Start Slowly:** If you decide to reintroduce foods, do so gradually. Start with one type of food at a time and pay close attention to how your body responds.

- **Keep a Food Journal:** Document the reintroduction process in a food journal. Record the foods you reintroduce, the portion sizes, and any symptoms or changes in how you feel.

- **Listen to Your Body:** Pay attention to your body's signals. If you experience digestive discomfort, inflammation, or other adverse effects when reintroducing specific foods, consider eliminating them again.

- **Focus on Low-Lectin Foods:** When reintroducing foods, opt for low-lectin options that are less likely to cause problems.

These might include well-cooked legumes, grains with lower lectin content, or nightshade vegetables without the skin or seeds.

long-term success on a lectin-free diet involves commitment, support, and potentially the gradual reintroduction of foods. By setting realistic expectations, finding support, and making informed choices about food reintroduction, you can make your dietary journey sustainable and beneficial for your health and well-being.

CHAPTER 9

Recipes and Meal Plans

9.1 Breakfast

Lectin-Free Scrambled Eggs with Spinach and Tomatoes:

Ingredients:

- 2 large eggs

- 1 cup fresh spinach leaves

- 1/2 cup cherry tomatoes, halved

- Salt and pepper to taste

- Olive oil for cooking

Instructions:

1. Heat a small amount of olive oil in a non-stick skillet over medium heat.

2. Add the cherry tomatoes and sauté until they begin to soften.

3. Add the fresh spinach and cook until wilted.

4. Beat the eggs in a bowl, season with salt and pepper, and pour them into the skillet with the vegetables.

5. Stir and cook until the eggs are scrambled and fully cooked.

6. Serve hot.

9.2 Lunch

Lectin-Free Quinoa Salad with Grilled Chicken:

Ingredients:

- 1 cup cooked quinoa
- Grilled chicken breast, sliced
- Cucumber, diced
- Red bell pepper, diced
- Red onion, finely chopped

- Fresh parsley, chopped

- Lemon vinaigrette dressing (lemon juice, olive oil, salt, and pepper)

Instructions:

1. In a large bowl, combine the cooked quinoa, diced cucumber, red bell pepper, red onion, and fresh parsley.

2. Top with sliced grilled chicken breast.

3. Drizzle with lemon vinaigrette dressing.

4. Toss to combine and serve as a refreshing, lectin-free lunch.

9.3 Dinner

Lectin-Free Baked Salmon with Roasted Asparagus:

Ingredients:

- Salmon fillets
- Asparagus spears
- Olive oil
- Lemon zest
- Garlic powder
- Salt and pepper to taste

Instructions:

1. Preheat the oven to 400°F (200°C).

2. Place salmon fillets on a baking sheet lined with parchment paper.

3. Drizzle olive oil over the salmon and season with lemon

zest, garlic powder, salt, and pepper.

4. Arrange asparagus spears around the salmon.

5. Drizzle olive oil over the asparagus and season with salt and pepper.

6. Bake for 15-20 minutes or until the salmon is cooked through and the asparagus is tender.

7. Serve the baked salmon and asparagus together.

9.4 Snacks and Desserts

Lectin-Free Guacamole:

Ingredients:

- Ripe avocados, mashed

- Diced tomatoes

- Chopped red onion

- Fresh cilantro, chopped

- Lime juice

- Salt and pepper to taste

Instructions:

1. In a bowl, combine the mashed avocados, diced tomatoes, chopped red onion, and fresh cilantro.

2. Squeeze fresh lime juice over the mixture and season with salt and pepper.

3. Mix well and serve as a delicious lectin-free snack with vegetable sticks or rice cakes.

Lectin-Free Berry Salad:

Ingredients:

- A mix of berries (e.g., strawberries, blueberries, raspberries)

- Fresh mint leaves, chopped

- A drizzle of balsamic vinegar (choose one without added sugar)

Instructions:

1. Wash and prepare the berries by cutting larger ones into bite-sized pieces.

2. Toss the berries together in a bowl.

3. Sprinkle with chopped fresh mint leaves.

4. Drizzle a small amount of balsamic vinegar (ensure it's lectin-free) for added flavor.

5. Gently mix and enjoy this naturally sweet and refreshing dessert.

9.5 Sample Meal Plans

Here are two sample lectin-free meal plans for a day:

Sample Meal Plan 1:

- **Breakfast:** Lectin-Free Scrambled Eggs with Spinach and Tomatoes

- **Lunch:** Lectin-Free Quinoa Salad with Grilled Chicken

- **Dinner:** Lectin-Free Baked Salmon with Roasted Asparagus

- **Snack:** Lectin-Free Guacamole with Vegetable Sticks

- **Dessert:** Lectin-Free Berry Salad with Balsamic Drizzle

Sample Meal Plan 2:

- **Breakfast:** Lectin-Free Smoothie (Blend almond milk, spinach, banana, and almond butter)

- **Lunch:** Mixed Green Salad with Grilled Shrimp (Lettuce, cucumber, avocado, grilled shrimp, and olive oil dressing)

- **Dinner:** Lectin-Free Stir-Fried Chicken with Broccoli (Chicken, broccoli, bell peppers, and coconut aminos)

- **Snack:** Sliced Cucumbers and Red Pepper with Hummus (lectin-free hummus)

- **Dessert:** Lectin-Free Coconut Milk Chia Pudding

These sample meal plans offer a variety of lectin-free options for breakfast, lunch, dinner, snacks, and desserts to help you get started on a lectin-free diet. Remember to adjust portion sizes and ingredients to suit your dietary preferences and calorie needs.